Baby Chronicles Pregnancy Planner

MW00683219

Month: Year:

Sunday	Monday	Tuesday	Wednesday	Thursday	Friday	Saturday	Week

Take your maternity multi-vitamins at night to avoid nausea

Month: Year:

Sunday	Monday	Tuesday	Wednesday	Thursday	Friday	Saturday	Week

Pick your baby's name carefully. It has to last a lifetime

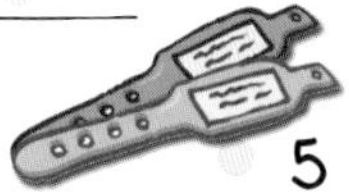

Month: Year:

Sunday	Monday	Tuesday	Wednesday	Thursday	Friday	Saturday	Week

An innie or outie belly button is not determined by the way the doctor cuts the umbilical cord

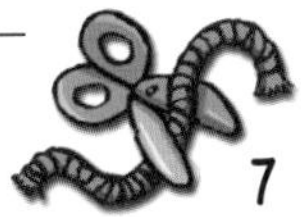

Month: Year:

Sunday	Monday	Tuesday	Wednesday	Thursday	Friday	Saturday	Week

There is no correlation between pregnancy weight gain, baby's birth weight and child's eventual weight

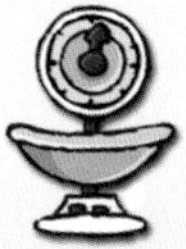

Month: Year:

Sunday	Monday	Tuesday	Wednesday	Thursday	Friday	Saturday	Week

A digital baby monitor is clearer and has less static and interference than an analog monitor

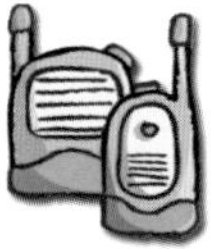

Month: Year:

Sunday	Monday	Tuesday	Wednesday	Thursday	Friday	Saturday	Week

When venturing outdoors, dress your baby as you would dress yourself, plus one layer

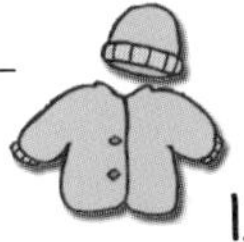

Month: Year:

Sunday	Monday	Tuesday	Wednesday	Thursday	Friday	Saturday	Week

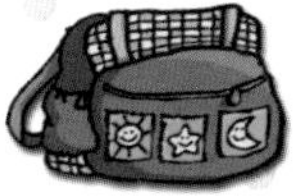

Keep extra diapers, wipes and disposable bags in your car

Month: Year:

Sunday	Monday	Tuesday	Wednesday	Thursday	Friday	Saturday	Week

Use cornstarch to absorb any pee that leaks onto the carpet

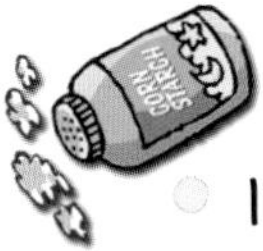

Month: Year:

Sunday	Monday	Tuesday	Wednesday	Thursday	Friday	Saturday	Week

Babies under 6 months of age should not use suntan lotion because the chemicals can get absorbed into their skin.

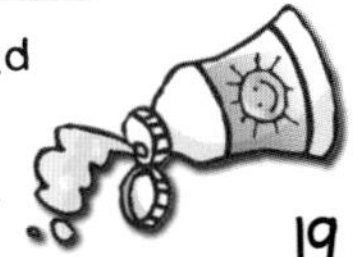

Month: Year:

Sunday	Monday	Tuesday	Wednesday	Thursday	Friday	Saturday	Week

To prevent dental problems, babies using pacifiers should be weaned off by 6 months of age

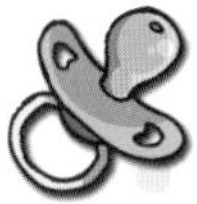

Month: Year:

Sunday	Monday	Tuesday	Wednesday	Thursday	Friday	Saturday	Week

Keep extra batteries on hand for your baby monitor and breast pump

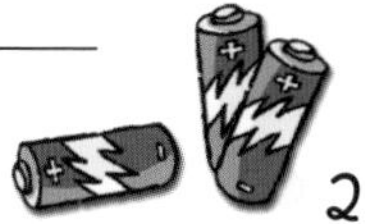

Month: Year:

Sunday	Monday	Tuesday	Wednesday	Thursday	Friday	Saturday	Week

Mineral oil loosens the wax build-up in kids' ears

Appointment Reminders and Details

Appt Date	Week	Your Blood Pr.	Your Weight	Baby's Heart Beat

Appt Date	Week	Your Blood Pr.	Your Weight	Baby's Heart Beat

Record your blood pressure, weight gain and your baby's heart beat.
In the "week" column, record how far along you are in your pregnancy.

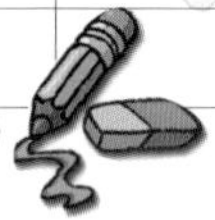

Am I Pregnant?

Every woman and every pregnancy is different. Some women may experience a few, all or none of the following signs of pregnancy. Always consult your physician.

Signs of Pregnancy

☑ Missed menstrual cycle
☑ Sustained high basal body temperature (BBT)
☑ A sensitivity to smells
☑ Food cravings
☑ Heartburn
☑ Nausea
☑ Constipation
☑ Bloating, backaches, and mood swings
☑ Tender or swollen breasts
☑ Darkening or broadening of the areola (area around nipple)
☑ Headaches
☑ Frequent urination

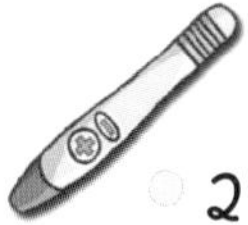

Important Tips Before and During Pregnancy

Follow these tips to increase the chances of a healthy baby and a healthy you.

Health Care

- ☑ Both you and your spouse/partner should take blood tests to determine blood incompatibilities and Rh factor
- ☑ Start on a prenatal vitamin containing iodine and folic acid *before* you are pregnant
  * Folic acid is especially important in the first trimester to lower your risk of some birth defects. Iodine is important for the fetus and baby to produce thyroid hormones. Record your vitamin intake using the rolling calendars (pages 2 - 25)
- ☑ Consult your physician before starting or stopping any medications
- ☑ Avoid x-rays, saunas, hot tubs, sun, lotions with chemicals and insect repellant
- ☑ Get plenty of sleep and find ways to control stress
- ☑ Wash hands frequently
- ☑ Stay away from second-hand smoke
- ☑ If you are nursing, continue taking prenatal vitamins even after your baby is born

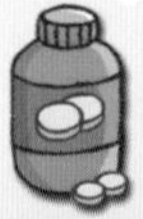

Food & Drink

- ☑ Eat healthy; drink lots of fluids to avoid dehydration; limit sugary fruit juices
- ☑ Limit caffeine
- ☑ Wash produce well; make sure your meat and fish are fresh and well-cooked
- ☑ Avoid nitrates & additives
- ☑ No alcohol, no artificial sweeteners

Other

- ☑ No smoking, no drugs
- ☑ Prescription drugs must be taken under your doctor's supervision
- ☑ Exercise. It is good for *you* and the baby (unless your doctor tells you otherwise)
- ☑ Look out for high blood pressure while pregnant
- ☑ Don't hesitate to discuss anything with your doctor and see your doctor regularly
- ☑ Get to know your body and listen to its signals

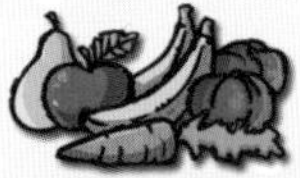

Reducing the Discomforts of Pregnancy

Morning Sickness

Morning sickness does not only happen in the morning; it can occur at any time during the day or night. The good news is that it *usually* stops by the end of the first trimester.

- ☑ Upon waking, get out of bed slowly. This gives your blood a chance to circulate
- ☑ Keep unsalted crackers and water next to your bed; crackers help relieve nausea and water helps you digest the crackers
- ☑ Eat small portions of food throughout the day because hunger can make nausea worse
- ☑ Try smaller, bland meals of carbohydrates (rice, potatoes). Make sure to get your protein
- ☑ Add higher protein foods to your diet (eggs, cheese, beans)
- ☑ Cut down on spicy, greasy, fried foods
- ☑ Avoid smells that you find unpleasant
- ☑ Lie down when you feel the first signs of nausea coming on

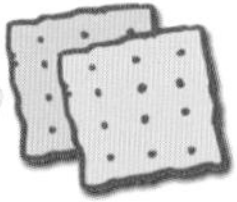

Heartburn

One of the primary reasons women develop heartburn during pregnancy is hormonal variations. Hormones can relax the valve that normally prevents stomach acid from backing up into the esophagus.

- ☑ To reduce heartburn in the day, avoid tight clothing
- ☑ To reduce heartburn at night, sleep with head elevated
- ☑ Avoid bending down using your back, instead bend at your knees
- ☑ Most antacids are safe during pregnancy, but clear it with your doctor first

Back Pain

- ☑ Have your spouse/partner give you a gentle muscle massage
- ☑ Take a warm bath. The heat and water may relieve some of the pain
- ☑ Try a support pillow in bed. Sleep on your side with a wedge-shaped pillow placed under your belly

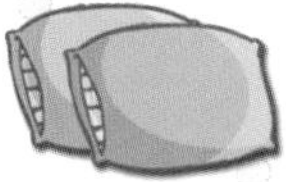

Exercising During Pregnancy

Should You or Shouldn't You Exercise?

- ☑ You should. Both you and your baby will benefit from exercise
- ☑ Exercise can help you look and feel better, prepare your body for birth by making it easier to adapt to changes in your body and, after birth, can help you regain your pre-pregnancy body more quickly
- ☑ Exercise may also reduce the risk of gestational diabetes, reduce discomforts like backache, constipation, fatigue, bloating and swelling

Getting Started

- ☑ Consult your doctor before beginning any exercise program
- ☑ Start gradually
- ☑ Dress comfortably in loose-fitting clothes and wear a support bra
- ☑ Stay hydrated by drinking plenty of water
- ☑ Skip your exercises if you are sick
- ☑ Always listen to your body

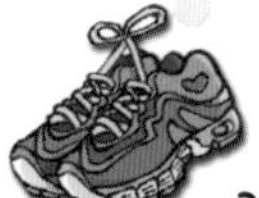

Recommended Exercises

For cardiovascular exercise, try ...

- ☑ Swimming
- ☑ Walking
- ☑ Aerobic activity at half of your pre-pregnancy level

For stress reduction and mental well-being, try yoga. Focus on ...

- ☑ Back muscles - to improve strength and posture, and to lessen the strain of pregnancy on your lower back
- ☑ Abdominal muscles - to make it easier to carry the growing weight of the baby, and to have extra strength when pushing during labor
- ☑ Pelvic muscles - practice Kegel exercises to allow the vagina to widen more easily during delivery and to correct bladder control problems

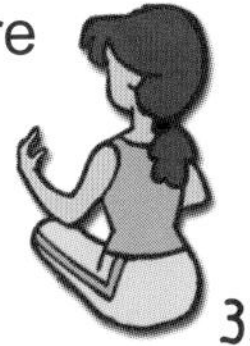

Exercising During Pregnancy

Exercises to Avoid

☑ No contact sports. Try to avoid falling
☑ No exercises that require you to lie flat on your back. Avoid pressure on the lungs and arteries
☑ No jarring or leaping activities. Avoid bouncing the fetus

Certain physical conditions preclude any form of exercise:

☑ Women experiencing high-risk pregnancies, second or third trimester bleeding, or heart disease should not exercise
☑ Women with severe anemia, poorly controlled high blood pressure or Type 1 diabetes and obesity are cautioned to speak with their doctor
☑ Women with no history of exercise should speak with their doctor and begin gradually

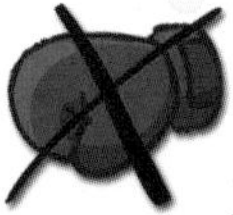

Important Information on Breast Feeding

- ☑ Breastfed babies need a vitamin D supplement beginning at one month of age. Discuss with your doctor
- ☑ Expressed milk can last 24 hours in the refrigerator and up to a month in the freezer
- ☑ To avoid the loss of nutrients, frozen or refrigerated expressed milk should not be reheated in the microwave. Instead, warm or melt the frozen milk by running the bottle under hot water
- ☑ When expressing milk, try to express at the same time every day, to get a regular flow going
- ☑ To avoid muscle and backache when nursing, use a nursing pillow or prop your arms up with a regular pillow
- ☑ Investigate breast feeding resources in your area

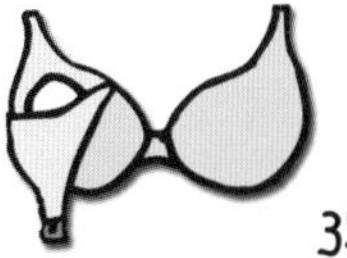

Important Information on Bottle Feeding

- ☑ Always test the temperature of formula or food that is warmed up because a baby's palette can easily burn
- ☑ Some babies display minor forms of lactose intolerance in the first year. Consult your doctor and discuss switching from cow-based to soy-based formula. This type of allergy often disappears after the child reaches one year of age
- ☑ Follow directions on the formula container to ensure that you are getting the correct water-to-powder ratio
- ☑ Avoid bottles manufactured with bisphenol A (BPA)
- ☑ Opt for a clear silicone nipple over latex rubber nipples
- ☑ Bottles and nipples are dishwasher-safe if placed on the top rack
- ☑ Choose between ready-to-use formula (very convenient but more expensive), liquid formula (mix with sterilized water) and powdered formula (mix with sterilized water but sometimes difficult to dissolve)

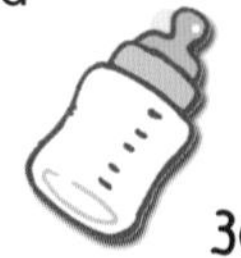

Baby Care Made Easier

- ☑ Baby's soft spot on the head (fontanelle) will close by about one and a half years of age
- ☑ Babies should have 4 to 6 wet diapers a day to ensure they are properly hydrated
- ☑ Messy diaper change? Change your baby in the crib so you can walk away to throw out the diaper without worrying about your baby rolling off a changing table
- ☑ Keep extra disposable garbage bags at the bottom of the diaper pail, underneath the bag currently being used. When you have to throw out a full bag of soiled diapers, another clean bag is readily available
- ☑ Diaper rash can be relieved by wiping baby's bottom clean with water, allowing baby's bottom to air dry and letting your baby go without a diaper. Keep your baby on a thick towel to avoid a mess on the floor
- ☑ When changing a boy's diaper, place a clean wash cloth over the groin area to avoid a surprise baby shower

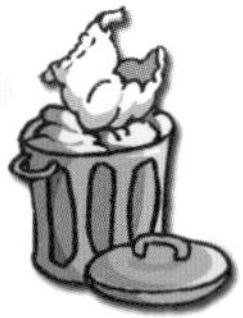

Baby Care Made Easier

- ☑ Keep extra baby wipes in different areas of the house and in the car. It is an easy way to clean up after your baby
- ☑ Keep extra diapers around the house, in every room and in the car
- ☑ Place a receiving blanket over your baby's crib sheet so if the diaper leaks, you don't have to change the whole bed
- ☑ Line the crib with a disposable mattress pad to protect the bed from diaper leaks
- ☑ If your baby has a cold or is congested, raise the crib angle by placing a folded towel under the mattress at your baby's head and use a cold-air humidifier
- ☑ Keep a change of clothes in the car for surprise diaper accidents
- ☑ Consider investing in a convertible stroller/car seat so as not to disturb baby when moving between car and other activities

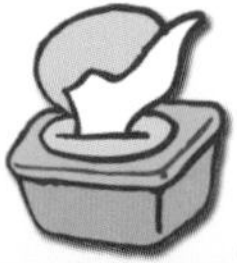

Making Your Home Baby Safe

A home must be baby-proofed to be a safe and happy haven for an infant under 6 months.

Baby's Room

- ☑ Cribs have to meet current standards to be safe. If you are buying a used crib, ensure the slats are no more than 2.4 inches (6 cms) apart and that none of the crib slats are broken or missing
- ☑ Never locate your baby's crib near a window, venetian blinds, or under a picture or wall-hanging
- ☑ Consider using cordless window coverings
- ☑ Don't use tacks or staples to secure items to the wall because these can fall out and be swallowed
- ☑ Crib sheets, sleepwear and blankets should be fire-resistant
- ☑ Don't leave a baby with a bottle in a crib. Among other things, extensive bottle use can lead to ear and teeth problems

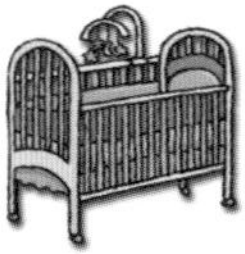

Making Your Home Baby Safe

Baby's Room

☑ Crib rails should always be raised and locked into their closed position. You never know when your baby will venture over the side

☑ Never leave your baby alone on a bed or diaper-changing table

Bathtime

☑ Always test the bath water temperature *before* immersing your baby in the bath. Also, make sure your hot water heater is set at a reasonable level

☑ Never leave your baby unattended in a bathtub, not even for a second

☑ Never leave a bathtub or bucket filled with water unattended because babies can fall in and drown

☑ Never answer the phone while your baby is in the bath

☑ As an alternative to a baby bath tub, consider using a bath sling or a foam bathtub insert that fits inside a regular bath tub

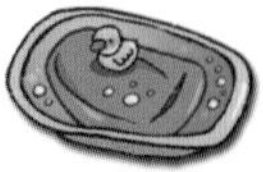

Arming Your House

- ☑ Have a fire extinguisher on each level of your home and know how to use it. Keep it easily accessible but *away* from the stove
- ☑ Install smoke detectors on each level of your home
- ☑ Install carbon monoxide detectors on each level of your home
- ☑ When adjusting clocks for Daylight Saving Time (DST), change batteries in smoke and carbon monoxide detectors
- ☑ Keep a first-aid kit in your house. Everyone should know where it is kept, including the babysitter
- ☑ Enroll in a first aid and CPR course
- ☑ Keep extra batteries on hand for baby monitors, electric swings, mobiles ....
- ☑ Install window guards on upper level windows

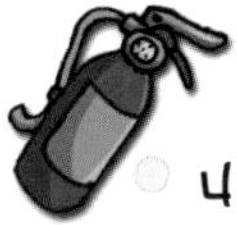

Making Your Car Baby Safe

Much of a baby's days are spent travelling around in a car. Choose a car seat that is effective, easy-to-use and is the right size for your child.

- ☑ Newborns up to 20 lbs (9 kg) must be secured in a rear-facing infant carrier, placed in the back seat of a car
- ☑ Children weighing between 20 to 40 lbs (9 to 18 kgs), who can sit up themselves, should be placed in a forward-facing car seat, preferably in the back seat of the car
- ☑ Ensure car seats are properly secured, tethered and lock-clipped
- ☑ Know how to use your car seat
- ☑ Avoid using old or second-hand car seats. If you must use a second-hand seat, make sure it has the original instructions (or contact the manufacturer for a replacement copy), has all its parts (check the manual), has never been involved in a serious accident, and hasn't been recalled
- ☑ Use a neck hugger to prevent your baby's head from bouncing around

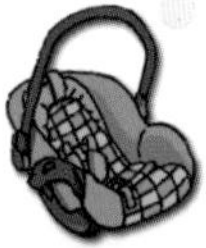

- ☑ Install an infant car mirror designed for infants sitting in rear-facing car seats. It allows you to safely keep an eye on your baby while you are driving
- ☑ Never place a child, 12 years and under, in a passenger seat equipped with an air bag
- ☑ New laws have come into effect regarding child car safety and booster seats. Learn about them
- ☑ Never drive in a car with a baby on your lap
- ☑ Your local police or fire stations often offer free child safety seat installation and inspection

Safety Seat Checklist

- ☑ Have I read the label on the safety belt and seat for any special instructions?
- ☑ Is my baby in the back seat?
- ☑ Is my baby facing the rear of the car?
- ☑ Does the safety belt or special anchor hold the child safety seat tightly in place?
- ☑ Does the harness fit snugly around my baby?
- ☑ Does my baby's head have support?

Must-Haves for Any Home with Babies

Safety, Health & First Aid	Parent Stuff
Baby thermometer	Infant car seat
Nose aspirator, baby nail clippers	Baby monitor
Baby acetaminophen	Cordless phone
Smoke and carbon monoxide detectors	Baby Chronicles, My Very Own Story
Fire extinguisher	Camera and videocamera
First-aid kit	Stroller
Chimes that sound when door / window opens	Extra batteries for the above electronics

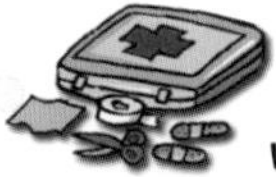

Handy Telephone Numbers

Name	Phone No.

Name	Phone No.

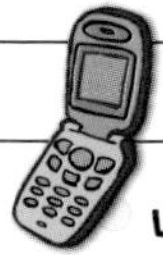

Mom's Medical Information

Doctor (OBGyn)			
Telephone No.		Address	
Important Information			
Doctor (GP)			
Telephone No.		Address	
Important Information			
Hospital (Delivery)			
Telephone No.		Address	
Important Information			
Pharmacy			
Telephone No.		Address	
Other			

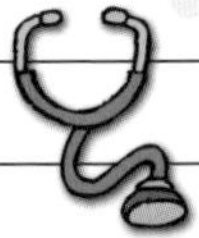

Baby's Medical Information

Doctor (Pediatrician)			
Telephone No.		Address	
Important Information			
Hospital (Children's)			
Telephone No.		Address	
Important Information			
Pharmacy			
Telephone No.		Address	
Other			

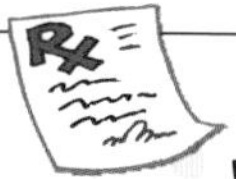

Personal Information

Name			
Address			
Home Phone No.		Cell Phone No.	
Work Place Name		Work Place No.	
Work Place Address			
Health Card No.			
Blood Type		Allergies	

	Name	Home Phone No.	Cell No.
Spouse/partner			
Babysitter			
Grandma			
Friend			

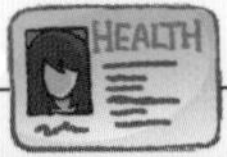

Notes

Notes

Baby Chronicles Registry

Please register as a member of the Baby Chronicles family. We will keep you informed of new product developments.

Name ______________________________ Date ____________________

Street ____________________________ City ______________________

State/Province __________ Country __________ Zip/Postal Code __________

Phone # (   )_______________ E-mail ____________________________

Name of store where Baby Chronicles Pregnancy Planner was purchased / or gift ____________________

To help us better understand you, would you please fill in this brief questionnaire? Thank you!

1. How old are you? Circle age range. 18 - 24 25 - 35 35+
2. Occupation: ______________________________
3. Do you have Baby Chronicles and School Year Chronicles? Yes or No. If yes, circle the ones you have.
4. Comments / suggestions: ____

____

____

Stamp
Me

Kiddy Chronicles Publishing
1057 Steeles Avenue West, P.O. Box 81512
Toronto, Ontario, Canada
M2R 3X1

BCPP-2010-1

Notes

2010

January

S	M	T	W	T	F	S
					1	2
3	4	5	6	7	8	9
10	11	12	13	14	15	16
17	18	19	20	21	22	23
24	25	26	27	28	29	30
31						

February

S	M	T	W	T	F	S
	1	2	3	4	5	6
7	8	9	10	11	12	13
14	15	16	17	18	19	20
21	22	23	24	25	26	27
28						

March

S	M	T	W	T	F	S
	1	2	3	4	5	6
7	8	9	10	11	12	13
14	15	16	17	18	19	20
21	22	23	24	25	26	27
28	29	30	31			

April

S	M	T	W	T	F	S
				1	2	3
4	5	6	7	8	9	10
11	12	13	14	15	16	17
18	19	20	21	22	23	24
25	26	27	28	29	30	

May

S	M	T	W	T	F	S
						1
2	3	4	5	6	7	8
9	10	11	12	13	14	15
16	17	18	19	20	21	22
23	24	25	26	27	28	29
30	31					

June

S	M	T	W	T	F	S
		1	2	3	4	5
6	7	8	9	10	11	12
13	14	15	16	17	18	19
20	21	22	23	24	25	26
27	28	29	30			

July

S	M	T	W	T	F	S
				1	2	3
4	5	6	7	8	9	10
11	12	13	14	15	16	17
18	19	20	21	22	23	24
25	26	27	28	29	30	31

August

S	M	T	W	T	F	S
1	2	3	4	5	6	7
8	9	10	11	12	13	14
15	16	17	18	19	20	21
22	23	24	25	26	27	28
29	30	31				

September

S	M	T	W	T	F	S
			1	2	3	4
5	6	7	8	9	10	11
12	13	14	15	16	17	18
19	20	21	22	23	24	25
26	27	28	29	30		

October

S	M	T	W	T	F	S
					1	2
3	4	5	6	7	8	9
10	11	12	13	14	15	16
17	18	19	20	21	22	23
24	25	26	27	28	29	30
31						

November

S	M	T	W	T	F	S
	1	2	3	4	5	6
7	8	9	10	11	12	13
14	15	16	17	18	19	20
21	22	23	24	25	26	27
28	29	30				

December

S	M	T	W	T	F	S
			1	2	3	4
5	6	7	8	9	10	11
12	13	14	15	16	17	18
19	20	21	22	23	24	25
26	27	28	29	30	31	

2011

January

S	M	T	W	T	F	S
						1
2	3	4	5	6	7	8
9	10	11	12	13	14	15
16	17	18	19	20	21	22
23	24	25	26	27	28	29
30	31					

February

S	M	T	W	T	F	S
		1	2	3	4	5
6	7	8	9	10	11	12
13	14	15	16	17	18	19
20	21	22	23	24	25	26
27	28					

March

S	M	T	W	T	F	S
		1	2	3	4	5
6	7	8	9	10	11	12
13	14	15	16	17	18	19
20	21	22	23	24	25	26
27	28	29	30	31		

April

S	M	T	W	T	F	S
					1	2
3	4	5	6	7	8	9
10	11	12	13	14	15	16
17	18	19	20	21	22	23
24	25	26	27	28	29	30

May

S	M	T	W	T	F	S
1	2	3	4	5	6	7
8	9	10	11	12	13	14
15	16	17	18	19	20	21
22	23	24	25	26	27	28
29	30	31				

June

S	M	T	W	T	F	S
			1	2	3	4
5	6	7	8	9	10	11
12	13	14	15	16	17	18
19	20	21	22	23	24	25
26	27	28	29	30		

July

S	M	T	W	T	F	S
					1	2
3	4	5	6	7	8	9
10	11	12	13	14	15	16
17	18	19	20	21	22	23
24	25	26	27	28	29	30
31						

August

S	M	T	W	T	F	S
	1	2	3	4	5	6
7	8	9	10	11	12	13
14	15	16	17	18	19	20
21	22	23	24	25	26	27
28	29	30	31			

September

S	M	T	W	T	F	S
				1	2	3
4	5	6	7	8	9	10
11	12	13	14	15	16	17
18	19	20	21	22	23	24
25	26	27	28	29	30	

October

S	M	T	W	T	F	S
						1
2	3	4	5	6	7	8
9	10	11	12	13	14	15
16	17	18	19	20	21	22
23	24	25	26	27	28	29
30	31					

November

S	M	T	W	T	F	S
		1	2	3	4	5
6	7	8	9	10	11	12
13	14	15	16	17	18	19
20	21	22	23	24	25	26
27	28	29	30			

December

S	M	T	W	T	F	S
				1	2	3
4	5	6	7	8	9	10
11	12	13	14	15	16	17
18	19	20	21	22	23	24
25	26	27	28	29	30	31

2012

January

S	M	T	W	T	F	S
1	2	3	4	5	6	7
8	9	10	11	12	13	14
15	16	17	18	19	20	21
22	23	24	25	26	27	28
29	30	31				

February

S	M	T	W	T	F	S
			1	2	3	4
5	6	7	8	9	10	11
12	13	14	15	16	17	18
19	20	21	22	23	24	25
26	27	28	29			

March

S	M	T	W	T	F	S
				1	2	3
4	5	6	7	8	9	10
11	12	13	14	15	16	17
18	19	20	21	22	23	24
25	26	27	28	29	30	31

April

S	M	T	W	T	F	S
1	2	3	4	5	6	7
8	9	10	11	12	13	14
15	16	17	18	19	20	21
22	23	24	25	26	27	28
29	30					

May

S	M	T	W	T	F	S
		1	2	3	4	5
6	7	8	9	10	11	12
13	14	15	16	17	18	19
20	21	22	23	24	25	26
27	28	29	30	31		

June

S	M	T	W	T	F	S
					1	2
3	4	5	6	7	8	9
10	11	12	13	14	15	16
17	18	19	20	21	22	23
24	25	26	27	28	29	30

July

S	M	T	W	T	F	S
1	2	3	4	5	6	7
8	9	10	11	12	13	14
15	16	17	18	19	20	21
22	23	24	25	26	27	28
29	30	31				

August

S	M	T	W	T	F	S
			1	2	3	4
5	6	7	8	9	10	11
12	13	14	15	16	17	18
19	20	21	22	23	24	25
26	27	28	29	30	31	

September

S	M	T	W	T	F	S
						1
2	3	4	5	6	7	8
9	10	11	12	13	14	15
16	17	18	19	20	21	22
23	24	25	26	27	28	29
30						

October

S	M	T	W	T	F	S
	1	2	3	4	5	6
7	8	9	10	11	12	13
14	15	16	17	18	19	20
21	22	23	24	25	26	27
28	29	30	31			

November

S	M	T	W	T	F	S
				1	2	3
4	5	6	7	8	9	10
11	12	13	14	15	16	17
18	19	20	21	22	23	24
25	26	27	28	29	30	

December

S	M	T	W	T	F	S
						1
2	3	4	5	6	7	8
9	10	11	12	13	14	15
16	17	18	19	20	21	22
23	24	25	26	27	28	29
30	31					

2013

January

S	M	T	W	T	F	S
		1	2	3	4	5
6	7	8	9	10	11	12
13	14	15	16	17	18	19
20	21	22	23	24	25	26
27	28	29	30	31		

February

S	M	T	W	T	F	S
					1	2
3	4	5	6	7	8	9
10	11	12	13	14	15	16
17	18	19	20	21	22	23
24	25	26	27	28		

March

S	M	T	W	T	F	S
					1	2
3	4	5	6	7	8	9
10	11	12	13	14	15	16
17	18	19	20	21	22	23
24	25	26	27	28	29	30
31						

April

S	M	T	W	T	F	S
	1	2	3	4	5	6
7	8	9	10	11	12	13
14	15	16	17	18	19	20
21	22	23	24	25	26	27
28	29	30				

May

S	M	T	W	T	F	S
			1	2	3	4
5	6	7	8	9	10	11
12	13	14	15	16	17	18
19	20	21	22	23	24	25
26	27	28	29	30	31	

June

S	M	T	W	T	F	S
						1
2	3	4	5	6	7	8
9	10	11	12	13	14	15
16	17	18	19	20	21	22
23	24	25	26	27	28	29
30						

July

S	M	T	W	T	F	S
	1	2	3	4	5	6
7	8	9	10	11	12	13
14	15	16	17	18	19	20
21	22	23	24	25	26	27
28	29	30	31			

August

S	M	T	W	T	F	S
				1	2	3
4	5	6	7	8	9	10
11	12	13	14	15	16	17
18	19	20	21	22	23	24
25	26	27	28	29	30	31

September

S	M	T	W	T	F	S
1	2	3	4	5	6	7
8	9	10	11	12	13	14
15	16	17	18	19	20	21
22	23	24	25	26	27	28
29	30					

October

S	M	T	W	T	F	S
		1	2	3	4	5
6	7	8	9	10	11	12
13	14	15	16	17	18	19
20	21	22	23	24	25	26
27	28	29	30	31		

November

S	M	T	W	T	F	S
					1	2
3	4	5	6	7	8	9
10	11	12	13	14	15	16
17	18	19	20	21	22	23
24	25	26	27	28	29	30

December

S	M	T	W	T	F	S
1	2	3	4	5	6	7
8	9	10	11	12	13	14
15	16	17	18	19	20	21
22	23	24	25	26	27	28
29	30	31				

Baby Chronicles Pregnancy Planner

Product Listing	Prices
Baby Chronicles Pregnancy Planner	$ 9.95
Baby Chronicles, My Very Own Story	$19.95
School Year Chronicles: The Best of In-School and After-School	$19.95
JR & HIGH SCHOOL *Chronicles*, Knock Before Entering	$19.95
Les chroniques de Bébé: Mon histoire à moi	$19.95
LES CHRONIQUES DES ANNÉES D'ÉCOLE: LES MEILLEURS MOMENTS DE L'ÉCOLE ET D'APRÈS L'ÉCOLE	$19.95
Crónicas del Bebé, Historia de mi infancia	$19.95

We are always updating our product line to meet the needs of our customers.
Please visit us at www.babychronicles.com to see what is new and exciting and to order additional products.

Stickers for your planner

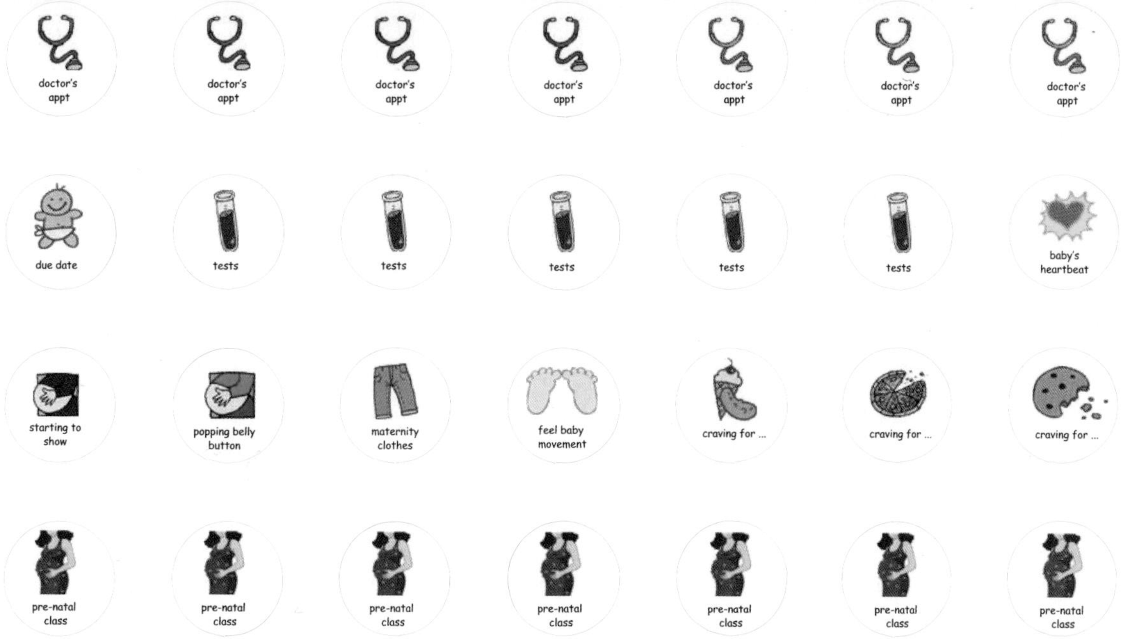

Stickers for your planner

- Mom weigh-in
- Mom weigh-in
- Mom weigh-in
- sonogram
- sonogram
- sonogram
- hospital visit
- crib shopping
- baby's room ready
- packed hospital bag
- baby shower
- maternity leave
- labor pains
- baby's birth
- twins
- twins
- first car trip
- home from the hospital
- nursing
- first bottle
- first bath
- sucks thumb
- first smile
- first laugh
- walk in stroller
- walk in baby carrier

Stickers for your planner

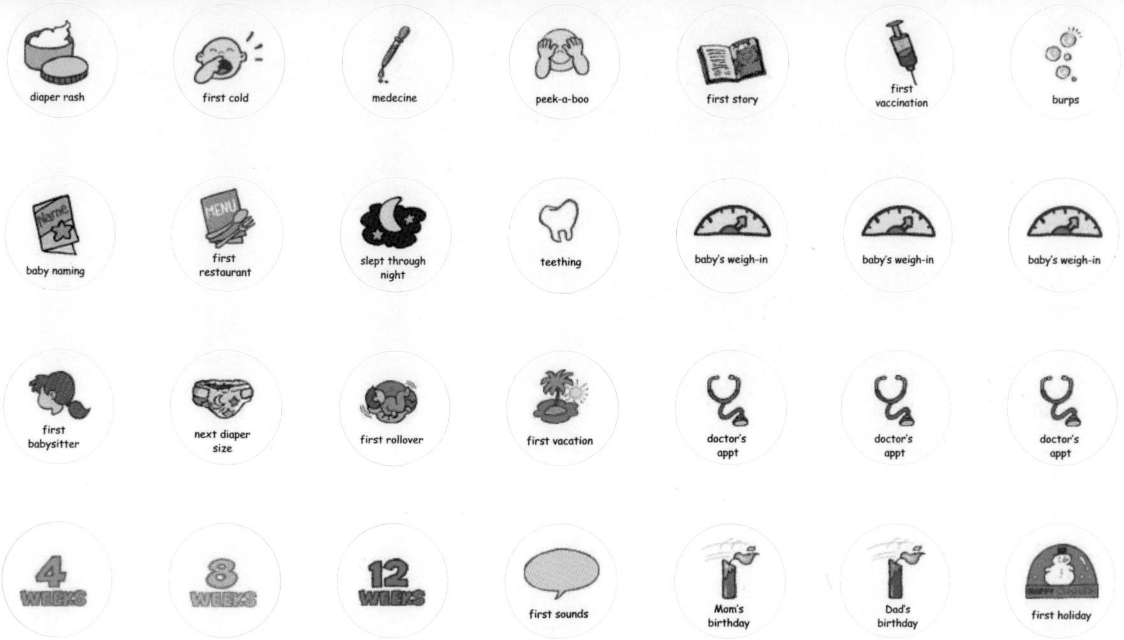